DK American College of Physicians

HOME MEDICAL GUIDE *to*

# MEMORY LOSS & DEMENTIA

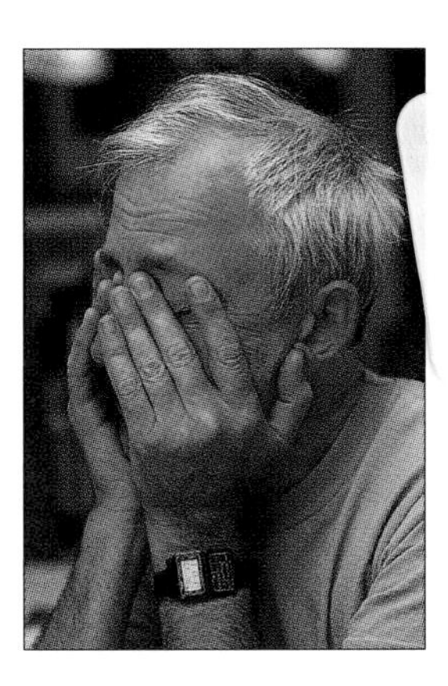



MEDICAL EDITOR
DAVID R. GOLDMANN, MD
ASSOCIATE MEDICAL EDITOR
DAVID A. HOROWITZ, MD

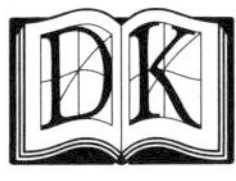


A DORLING KINDERSLEY BOOK

## Important

The American College of Physicians (ACP) Home Medical Guides provide general information on a wide range of health and medical topics. These books are not substitutes for medical diagnosis, and you should always consult your doctor on personal health matters before undertaking any program of therapy or treatment. Various medical organizations have different guidelines for diagnosis and treatment of the same conditions; the American College of Physicians–American Society of Internal Medicine (ACP–ASIM) has tried to present a reasonable consensus of these opinions.

Material in this book was reviewed by the ACP–ASIM for general medical accuracy and applicability in the United States; however, the information provided herein does not necessarily reflect the specific recommendations or opinions of the ACP–ASIM. The naming of any organization, product, or alternative therapy in these books is not an ACP–ASIM endorsement, and the omission of any such name does not indicate ACP–ASIM disapproval.

**DORLING KINDERSLEY**
LONDON, NEW YORK, AUCKLAND, DELHI,
JOHANNESBURG, MUNICH, PARIS, AND SYDNEY

DK www.dk.com

**Senior Editors** Jill Hamilton, Nicki Lampon
**Senior Designer** Jan English
**DTP Design** Jason Little
**Editor** Ashley Ren
**Medical Consultant** Stephen Arnold, MD

**Senior Managing Editor** Martyn Page
**Senior Managing Art Editor** Bryn Walls

Published in the United States in 2000 by
Dorling Kindersley Publishing, Inc.
95 Madison Avenue, New York, New York 10016

2 4 6 8 10 9 7 5 3 1



Based on an original work by Dr. Christopher Martyn and Dr. Catharine Gale.



Library of Congress Catalog Card Number 99-76851
ISBN 0-7894-5201-4

Reproduced by Colourscan, Singapore
Printed and bound in the United States by Quebecor World, Taunton, Massachusetts

# Contents

# I'm worried about my memory

*"I'm always forgetting people's names. Only last week I met someone who used to live just down the street. I knew exactly who she was, but I couldn't remember her name. It was so embarrassing. This is happening to me more and more often these days. And I worry about it. Is it going to get worse? Am I getting Alzheimer's disease or going senile?"*

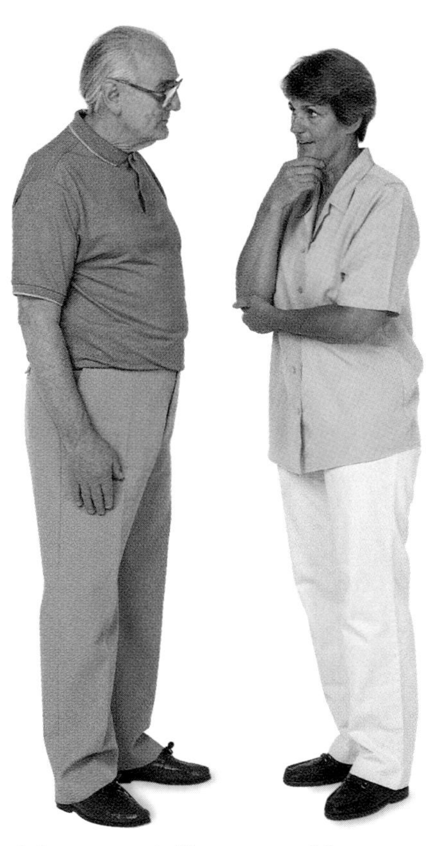

TROUBLE WITH NAMES
*Forgetting names is common with a failing memory, and meeting even familiar people may prove embarrassing.*

This sort of complaint is very common. Many people find that as they get older their memory seems to become less and less reliable. Perhaps, like the two people seen here in conversation, they meet someone whose face is familiar yet they are unable to remember his or her name.

The problem with memory is often most severe when it comes to remembering people's names. But people whose memory for names is unreliable may also be aware of lapses of memory of other things. They may find it difficult to remember appointments, tasks that need to be done, what to buy when shopping, or where they have put their keys or their glasses.

When slips of memory occur frequently, it is not surprising that people become worried. They may be afraid that they are becoming senile or beginning to develop Alzheimer's disease. While it is true that deterioration in memory can sometimes be an indication of something serious, there is often a much simpler explanation. If you or someone close to you is having trouble remembering things, we hope that the first three chapters in this book will help you understand what is going on, put the problem in proper perspective, and make it easier for you to cope.

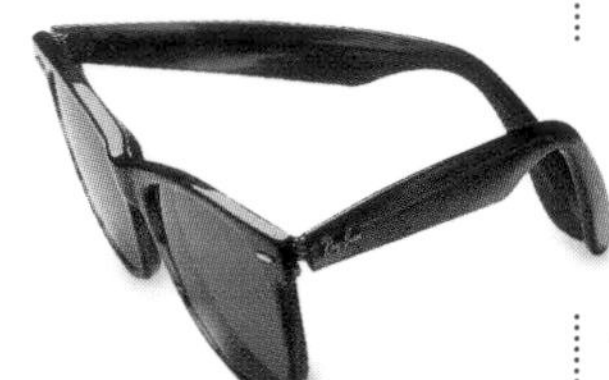

MISPLACING POSSESSIONS
*Forgetting where you have put things, such as your glasses, is an annoying and very common symptom of a deteriorating memory.*

## HOW MEMORY WORKS

Perhaps it would be helpful to start by explaining something about how memory works. Imagine that one morning a friend introduces you to a woman named Muriel Pritchett. Later that day, you bump into her again. "Hello, Muriel," you say. "We met this morning." It is obvious that you have remembered her name. But how?

Despite a great deal of scientific research, there is still much to be learned about the way memory works, but we already understand much about it. One way to think about memory is to divide its process into three stages.

### REGISTERING INFORMATION

The first stage of memory requires that you register the new information. When you were introduced to Muriel, you took note of her name and her face. Your brain absorbed this information and then transferred it to the part where memories are stored.

### Storing Information

During the second memory stage, your brain files away new information. You stored Muriel's name and appearance from the time of your first meeting until you encountered her again.

### Recalling Information

The third stage is the retrieval of this information from the part of the brain where it was stored. In our example, this stage occurred when you met Muriel for the second time and you were able to greet her by name.

All three stages must take place for your memory to work. If any of them had failed, you would have been unable to recall Muriel's name at your second meeting.

In many ways, the process is like putting a letter away in a filing cabinet so that you can refer to it in the future. Think of the letter as the new item of information. First, you have to realize that you may need it again. Second, you must store it in a safe place. And third, when you want to read it again, you have to open the right drawer of the filing cabinet and get it out. If you do not notice the importance of the letter in the first place or fail to file it correctly, you will not be able to find it when you need it again.

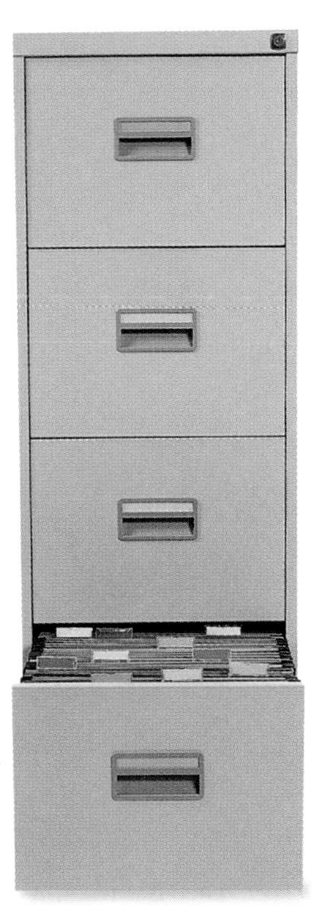

FILING INFORMATION
*Your brain acts as a filing cabinet, storing information until it is needed at some time in the future.*

## The Three Stages of Memory

- Register new information that is to be remembered.
- Store this information so that it can be retrieved.
- Retrieve it from storage when needed.

## TYPES OF MEMORY

Psychologists believe that there are several kinds of memory, each of which is used for storing different kinds of information. The part of our memory that we use for storing facts such as people's names is separate from the part that we use to store knowledge of how to do things. This explains why some people who have difficulty recalling the names of people they know well have no problem remembering how to use a can opener or turn on a television.

USEFUL FORGETTING
*Trivial information such as the items on the weekly shopping list is discarded quickly to avoid cluttering up your memory stores.*

## FORGETTING

We all forget things. Indeed, our memory could not work properly otherwise. Forgetting can be a useful process in which information that is no longer important is discarded. It would not be sensible to clutter your brain with memories of everything you bought in the supermarket last week, for example. Your brain makes decisions all the time about what to remember and what to forget. It stores what it considers to be important and discards what it thinks is trivial. However, everyone's brain makes mistakes occasionally, and sometimes things that are significant are forgotten.

All memories tend to fade as time passes. Facts used every day stay in the memory, while items of information that are seldom needed are harder to recall. For example, most people can remember their own telephone number. However, if they need to call the doctor, they have to look up the number in the phone book.

Recalling a fact or an event keeps that particular memory fresh and makes it easier to remember on future occasions. Conversely, facts that are never used will be gradually forgotten. For example, how many dates can you still remember from the history classes you took at school?

## WHAT AFFECTS MEMORY?

The efficiency and accuracy of memory depend on the circumstances in which we are using it. As we explained earlier, to store a piece of information in our memory, we first have to pay sufficient attention to the information in order to register and absorb it.

All sorts of factors can interfere with this crucial first stage of memory. They may include the following.

### OVERLOAD

If we are confronted with too much information at one time, we may find it impossible to recall much of it later. At a social occasion, we meet lots of new people, but afterward it is often difficult to remember their names or much else about them. This is because there was so much information to take in that our capacity to register and store all of the new information was overloaded.

People who are very busy can often find themselves forgetting things simply because they have so much on their minds.

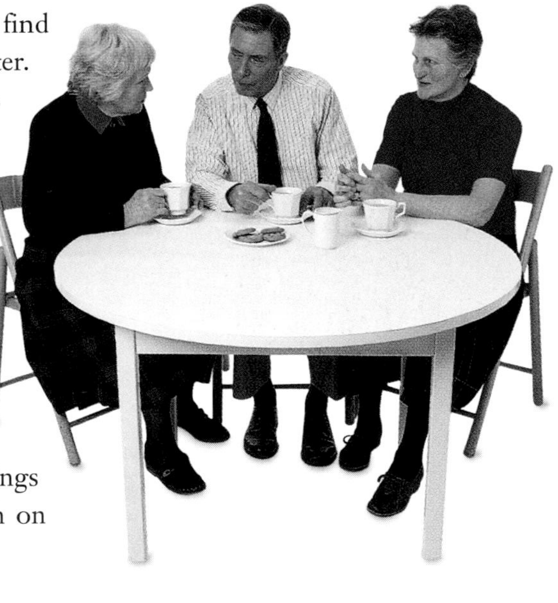

INFORMATION OVERLOAD
*Meeting new people, hearing their names, and listening to their conversation can be too much to take in, resulting in little being remembered.*

If a person's life follows a well-ordered routine, fewer demands are made on his or her memory than if it is varied and stressful.

### STATE OF MIND

For similar reasons, people who are anxious or depressed often find that their memory functions poorly. They become preoccupied by their inner thoughts and feelings and thus are too distracted to pay sufficient attention to new information. As a result, they do not register it properly.

EFFECTS OF ILLNESS
*Elderly people who have chronic physical illnesses such as a heart condition often have problems with their memory as well.*

### PHYSICAL DISABILITY

Older people whose hearing or vision is poor may have problems remembering things because their disabilities make it more difficult for them to register and absorb information.

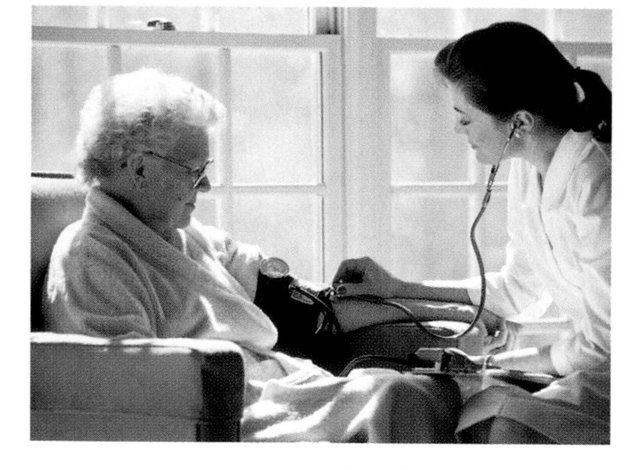

### ILLNESS

Physical illness, particularly in older people, can also have a damaging effect on mental functions. People who suffer from a chronic condition such as heart disease or diabetes may find that their thinking and their memory are not as good as they once were.

The precise reasons for this link between physical illness and memory function are not yet well understood, but the stresses of having to cope with illness, especially if the condition is painful, are bound to take their toll.

## THE IMPACT OF AGING

Every part of the body changes as we get older. Some of these changes begin quite early in life. Few athletes and sportsmen continue to break records after the age of 30 or so. Already their muscles, joints, hearts, and lungs are performing less well than they used to.

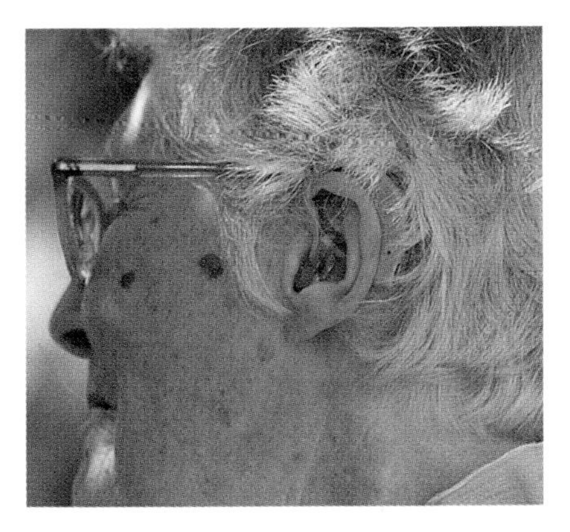

SOUND AND VISION
*Like memory, our hearing and eyesight commonly deteriorate as we advance into old age.*

Different parts of the body age faster than others, and individuals differ in which parts show the effects of age first. For instance, some elderly people develop osteoarthritis and need a hip replaced, while others become increasingly deaf and must wear a hearing aid.

### AGING AND MENTAL FUNCTIONS

It is important to realize that just as our bodies change as we get older, our mental processes change, too. Our reaction time tends to increase, and we process new information more slowly. Learning new things is more of a struggle for older people, especially if the information is presented too quickly or in an unfamiliar way. This is because older people tend to find it more difficult to divide their attention between two things and harder to ignore information that is irrelevant to the task at hand. As we get older, we become more concerned with accuracy than speed. This sometimes makes us slower when we carry out a job. However, aging is not all bad news. Research has shown that older people's greater experience may lead them to develop more efficient ways of doing things, which can outweigh the loss of speed. Indeed, old people often underestimate their own abilities.

## MEMORY AND AGE

Psychologists researching how mental functioning alters as we age have found that there is a gradual change in the way our memory works. One example of this is in the ability to remember a series of numbers for a short period of time. While young people are able to hold a sequence of seven or eight numbers in their heads for a minute or two, most people over the age of 60 or so can manage to retain a sequence of only five or six numbers. You may have noticed this yourself when you have been dialing a telephone number.

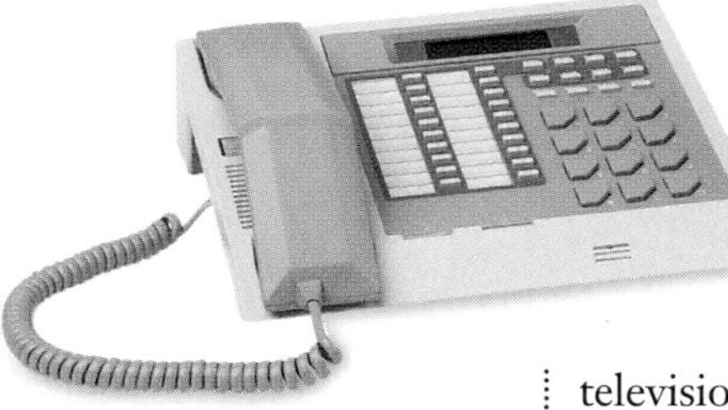

REMEMBERING NUMBERS
*As we get older, we find it increasingly difficult to retain long sequences of numbers, such as telephone numbers, in our heads.*

Our capacity to remember names seems to be especially vulnerable to the effects of age. When it comes to remembering factual information, such as what was said in a conversation, the contents of a radio or television program, or how to do something, most older people manage perfectly well.

Older people who are losing confidence in their ability to remember should take account of the fact that their memories contain much more than the memories of younger people. To go back to an earlier analogy, their filing cabinets are fuller. At the age of 70, the filing cabinets of memory contain information gathered over a period of time twice as long as that of a person aged 35. Looked at in this way, it is not surprising that older people are slower to retrieve memories and absorb new facts. Therefore, if you are worried about your memory, it makes sense to compare your performance with that of your contemporaries rather than with that of younger people.

## KEY POINTS

- The memory process can be divided into three stages: registering, storing, and recalling information.
- Everyone forgets things; our brains continually make decisions about what to forget and what to remember.
- Illness, anxiety, and information overload can affect our ability to remember.
- Most of us become more forgetful as we grow older.

# How well is your memory working?

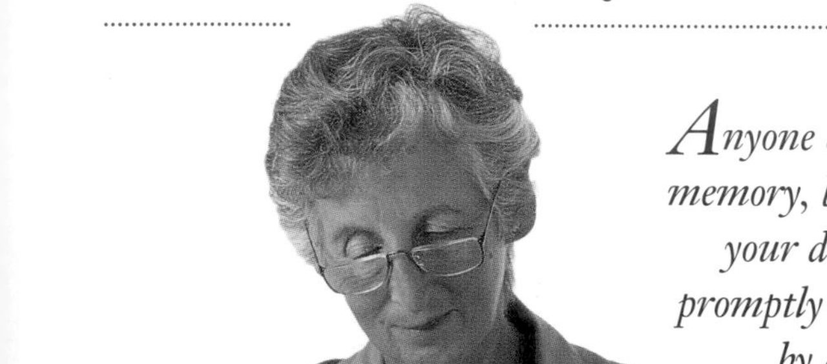

*Anyone can have occasional lapses of memory, but, if they occur frequently, your doctor should be informed promptly because they may be caused by a medical condition that is treatable. Gradual loss of short-term memory can affect a person in a variety of ways, some of which may limit your ability to live safely on your own.*

There are a variety of factors that are used to determine the condition of a person's memory and how it affects his or her ability to live independently. You can ask yourself specific questions if you are concerned about recent memory lapses. Other assessments should be made by a primary care physician or a specialist such as a geriatrician or psychologist.

Assessing Dependence
*Although memory lapses may be worrying, you may not know whether to consult a doctor. The answers to questions on memory loss and functional abilities may help in making an assessment.*

If either you or your family is concerned enough about your recent memory lapses to schedule an appointment with your doctor, the checkup is likely to consist of four basic parts: a detailed medical history, a physical examination (see What will your doctor do?, pp.41–47), a functional activities assessment (see p.18), and an examination of your mental status, which includes orientation, attention level, memory, and language skills.

## Questions to Assess your Memory

There are a number of questions that you can ask yourself, or your family can answer, in order to get an idea of whether your memory lapses might be serious.

- Do you often forget where you put things, lose objects at home, forget where things are normally kept, or look for them in the wrong place?
- Do you often fail to recognize places where you have been before?
- Do you often have to check that you have done something you meant to do?
- Do you often forget to take something with you when you go out?
- Do you often forget something you were told within the past couple of days?
- Do you often fail to recognize by sight close relatives and friends whom you see frequently?
- Do you often forget to pass on an important message or get the details mixed up or confused?
- Do you often forget important details about yourself, such as your date of birth, your address, or your telephone number?
- Do you often do some routine things twice, such as brushing your teeth or hair when you have just done so?

- Do you often repeat yourself when you are talking to someone, or ask him or her the same question twice?

## FUNCTIONAL ACTIVITIES

Certain activities are necessary for entirely independent living. A doctor or other medical professional can be helpful in determining whether you are or are not able to live independently and will make that recommendation based on your ability to carry out some of the following tasks. If you are totally dependent on someone else for at least three of the following activities, it is likely that you have a significant functional deficit.

- Writing checks, paying bills, or balancing a checkbook.
- Assembling tax records, business affairs, or papers.
- Shopping alone for clothes, household necessities, or groceries.
- Playing a game of skill or working on a hobby.
- Heating water, making a cup of coffee, or turning off the stove.
- Preparing a balanced meal.
- Keeping track of current events.
- Paying attention to, understanding, or discussing TV, books, and magazines.
- Remembering appointments, family occasions, holidays, or medications.
- Traveling out of the neighborhood, driving, or arranging to take public transportation.

## Key Points

- There are a variety of questions that can be used, some by patients or family members and others by medical professionals, to assess memory loss.
- Your ability to perform various functional activities without assistance will help determine your ability to live independently.

# How to cope with an unreliable memory

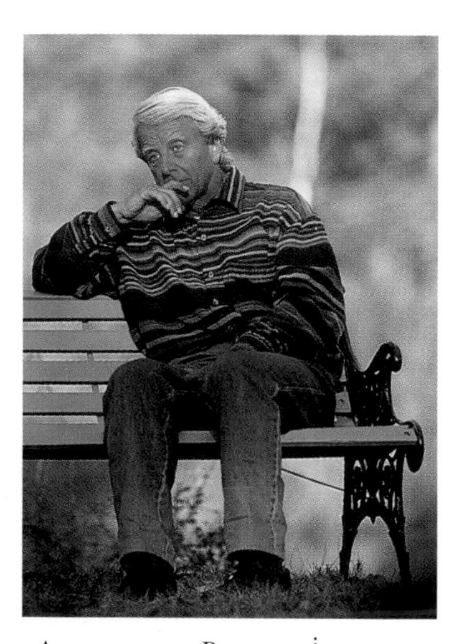

Admitting the Problem
*Being honest and recognizing that your memory is failing will help you come to terms with your problem.*

*Unfortunately, your memory is not a system like your heart and lungs for which "fitness" exercises can be prescribed. While mental stimulation is good, practice at memorizing information is very unlikely to improve your memory.*

However, there are a number of things you can do to make life easier, and this chapter offers some practical advice on how to cope.

## Assessing Yourself

The first step in coping with a memory that is becoming less reliable is admitting to yourself that you have a problem. The fact that you are reading this book probably indicates that you have already taken this step. We hope that you found the questions on pages 17 and 18 helpful. If so, you and your family should have reached an honest assessment of the state of your memory. It may not be as bad as you had feared.

The second important step is to understand what is happening. As we saw in the first chapter, everyone's memory deteriorates as he or she gets older, and you are not alone in experiencing this problem. Some people prefer to pretend to themselves that nothing is wrong, hoping that their memory problems will go away by themselves, but a positive attitude about dealing with your difficulties will prove much more advantageous.

## Being Honest

One extra problem that accompanies a failing memory is the embarrassment of forgetting names and faces or letting someone down. Under such circumstances, we sometimes try to disguise the fact that we have forgotten in order to save face. After all, it is quite possible to have a conversation with someone without using his or her name. Or we may try to avoid feelings of awkwardness by joking about our memory lapse, and a sense of humor certainly has its place in coping with the problems of a deteriorating memory.

If your forgetfulness is making life difficult for you, it is tempting to hide your anxiety behind a joke or to deflect attention from your predicament with a humorous remark, but this tactic may be unwise if it prevents you from tackling the problem in a serious way. Attempts to disguise the condition may, in the end, make life more difficult for you.

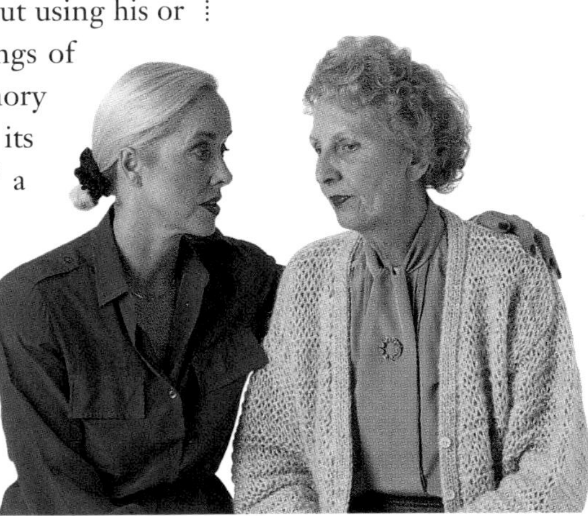

Family Support
*Discussing your problem with friends and family will often be a source of relief and help. They can offer emotional support and help remind you of important events and arrangements.*

Why not be honest and straightforward with your friends and relatives and tell them about the difficulties you are having? You will find that others often sympathize. They too are likely to have forgotten people's names, where they put things, or tasks that they were supposed to do.

### FINDING THE RIGHT WORDS

Sometimes it is hard to think of the right words to explain your problems. Try working out a few sentences in advance. Suppose you are worried that you might forget an arrangement to meet a friend. You could say something like "My memory is becoming rather unreliable. It would help if you could remind me."

Perhaps you are often faced with the awkward situation of being unable to remember someone's name. Later in this chapter we discuss ways to improve your memory of people's names, but, if despite all your efforts your mind is still a blank, do not be afraid to admit it. Say something like "I remember you very well, but I'm afraid I've forgotten your name!"

## FINDING WAYS TO COPE

There are a number of practical strategies you can adopt that will help make memory lapses less frequent. You probably use some memory aids already, such as an engagement book or a shopping list, but, if you feel that your memory is getting worse, or even if you just wish it were more reliable, it would be sensible to make greater use of them. Relying on such aids reduces the pressure on you to remember and will make you less anxious about forgetting. This in itself may make you less likely to forget things. As we explain later in this chapter, there are also a number of things you can do that may improve the way your memory stores information and make it easier to recall it later. Perhaps some of the ideas we recommend will seem too simple to be of much use, but give them a try anyway. Lots of people whose memories have been letting them down have found these strategies surprisingly helpful.

## Using Memory Prompts

If you discover that you are having problems remembering appointments and things you have to do, it may be helpful to try using some of the following memory prompts.

### Notes

Written notes are a simple but very effective reminder. Keep a notebook with you during the day so that you can write down all your tasks, particularly those that you cannot do immediately. These are the ones you are most likely to forget.

Try to get into the habit of making a note as soon as you think of something you have to do. Look at your notebook regularly, perhaps two or three times a day; there is no point in writing reminders to yourself unless you are going to see them frequently.

Some people find that when they are in bed at night they remember things they need to do the next day. It is a good idea to keep a paper and pen by your bed so that you can jot down these ideas when they occur to you.

Another way of prompting yourself is to put a note in a place where you cannot fail to see it. You can buy pads of brightly colored, sticky paper specially designed for leaving notes for yourself or other people. These are particularly useful if you have problems remembering to do something. For instance, if you need to take your coat to the cleaners, you could stick a note to yourself on the front door.

### Engagement and Wall Calendars

Engagement and wall calendars are also useful for reminding yourself to do things. Get into the habit of

Mark important dates

Keeping Appointments *Engagement and wall calendars are invaluable tools for helping you remember tasks and appointments. Keep them in prominent places.*

writing down all your appointments and all the things you need to do on a particular day. Put your calendar where you will see it several times a day, perhaps in the hall or the kitchen.

## Lists

Most people make shopping lists, especially when they have a lot to buy, but lists can be useful at other times, too. For instance, it can be helpful to make a list of things you need to talk about before you telephone someone.

When you are planning to go on vacation, make a list of everything you need to pack, check off each item as you pack it, and take a final look at the list again before you leave home.

## Medicine Organizers

If you need to remember to do something regularly and at particular times, such as taking pills, why not buy a watch that has an alarm, which can be set for certain times? Alternatively, you could opt for a special pill box with an alarm or one divided into compartments for each day of the week to make it easier to remember to take your daily dose and to check that you have taken it.

Another way of remembering to take your medication is to keep the pills near something that you use at about the time you should take them. For example, you could put the bottle of pills next to your toothbrush or beside the coffee pot. An established routine puts less stress on your memory, and you may find that if you regularly do things in a consistent order, you will do them almost automatically.

Remembering Medicines *If you need regular medication, use a special compartmentalized pill holder so that you can see when your medication is due at a glance.*

### Improving Your Memory for Tasks

On page 9, we explained that items of information are properly stored in your memory only if you pay attention to them. If you get into the habit of regularly thinking about the things you have to do, you are more likely to remember them. You may find it helpful to think about the tasks you do at certain times every day, such as when you start work or get back from lunch. This rehearsal of tasks helps keep them in your mind.

Sometimes you may find that you know there is something you need to do but cannot remember exactly what it is. In this situation, it can often help to go over other things you had to do to try to prompt your memory. For example, if you are out shopping you could think about all the other things you meant to buy. Or suppose there is a job in the yard you planned to do, but you have forgotten what it is. You could try thinking back to when you first thought about this particular task or go out to the yard and look around. Either of these actions will help stimulate your memory.

People often forget whether they have done a particular thing, such as shutting a window or turning off the oven. One way to help yourself remember is to talk aloud about what you are doing as you do it. So when you turn the oven off say, "I'm turning the oven off now." This concentrates your mind on what you are doing and helps fix it in your memory.

## Tips for Finding Things

It is all too easy to put down our glasses or keys somewhere around the house and then be unable to find them later. Or perhaps we buy something, put it away, and forget where it is.

## ORGANIZATION

Being well organized and keeping things in set places can help. Try to put things away in their proper places after you have used them. If you tend to misplace your keys around the house, you could put up a hook for them and get into the habit of hanging them there as soon as you come into the house.

## LISTS AND LABELS

It may also help to write a list of where you usually keep things and use it to make sure that you put things away in the right place. Labeling cabinets with a list of the contents is a good idea, too.

Self-adhesive labels with your name, address, and phone number are also useful if you have a tendency to leave things behind when you are out. Stick them on possessions such as your umbrella or bag. Then, if you do forget them, at least someone can return them to you.

## REMEMBERING WHERE SOMETHING IS

When you put something away, make a deliberate effort to concentrate on the particular place where you are putting it. Is there a reason why you are putting it in that particular place? You may find that saying aloud where you are putting something as you do it helps fix it in your memory. Forming a connection between the object and the place where you are putting it also helps you remember it later. For example, when you leave your car in a parking lot, concentrate on the position of the car in relation to the parking meter or the exit. After you have walked away from the car, picturing it and its position in the parking lot will help you store the memory properly.

If you do forget where you put something, go back in your mind to when you last remember having it. What were you doing? Then think what you did subsequently and where you were. Alternatively, think of all the places where you were likely to have put it.

## Remembering Names

When you meet someone for the first time, pay close attention to his or her name. If it is an unusual one, ask how it is spelled. As you talk to the person, use his or her name: "Where do you live, Muriel?" Repeating someone's name in conversation is a friendly thing to do, and the more attention you pay to the name, the more likely it is to become fixed in your memory. When you say goodbye, use the name again.

If someone's name is on the tip of your tongue, try going through the alphabet letter by letter or think of where you first heard the name. This might help you remember, but, if you still cannot recall the name, do not be afraid to admit it. It is a very common problem!

## Key Points

- Admitting that you have a problem is the first step in coping with an unreliable memory.
- Tell your friends and family that you are having difficulty with your memory.
- To help you remember where things are, decide on a particular place for articles that you frequently misplace and label cabinets and drawers.

# A sign of something serious?

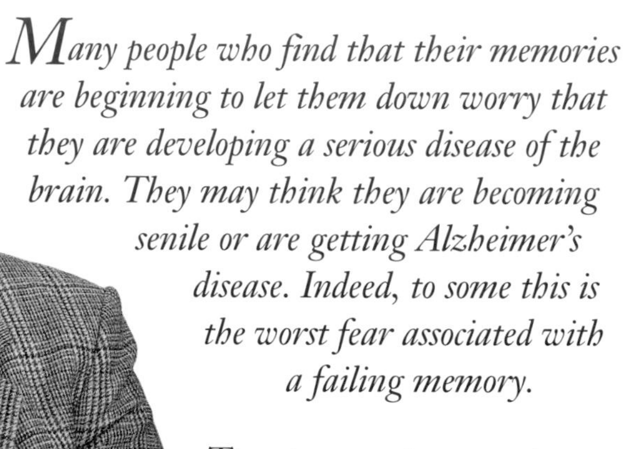

*Many people who find that their memories are beginning to let them down worry that they are developing a serious disease of the brain. They may think they are becoming senile or are getting Alzheimer's disease. Indeed, to some this is the worst fear associated with a failing memory.*

MENTAL DETERIORATION
*Although an unreliable memory is often the result of the normal aging process, occasionally, as in Ralph's case, it is a sign of something more serious, such as dementia.*

The inconvenience and acute embarrassment that result from a poor memory may worry people far less than the fear that their increasing memory lapses are a warning of approaching senility or dementia. They feel that they could cope with their memory problems as long as they knew that they were not going to become demented.

In the first part of this book, we described the normal changes in memory capacity that occur as we get older. We pointed out that an increasing number of memory lapses is simply something you have to learn to live with. However, sometimes changes in mental functions are a sign that something more serious than simple aging is occurring in the brain. In the next few pages, we discuss the sorts of things that indicate that you or the person you are worried about should see a doctor.

Case History: **DEMENTIA**

Ralph Emerson had retired from his job at the town hall a few months before his 65th birthday. At first, he and his wife, Lydia, had been busy doing all the things they had always promised themselves they would do when they had time. Ralph repainted the house, and Lydia made new curtains. They kept fit by swimming twice each week and took up new hobbies. Lydia discovered that she had a talent for watercolors, and Ralph taught himself to make frames for her pictures. They went on vacation together to places they had always wanted to visit, and one winter they went to visit their oldest daughter and her family in California. For a few years, Lydia thought that she had never known Ralph to be so happy. Gradually, however, she became aware that he was not his usual self.

Since retirement, it had become Ralph's habit to do the weekly shopping. Lydia had been delighted to have someone take over a chore that she had never liked. Ralph enjoyed it, taking pride in getting the best values and showing off his bargains with pleasure to his wife when he returned. But over the past few months, he seemed to have become a spendthrift.

On several occasions, he had come home with too many vegetables and expensive cuts of meat that were too big for the two of them to eat. Once he had bought cans of cat food, although they did not have a cat. He also began to forget things, despite Lydia's shopping list.

Lydia decided that she needed to go to the supermarket with him. They did their shopping and lined up at the checkout. When it was time to pay, Ralph got out his wallet. But he looked unsure of what to do next. Lydia was shocked to see that Ralph couldn't figure out how much money to give the cashier. She had to count out the bills herself.

Ralph began to change in other ways, too. He had always been a good-natured man even when he had been under pressure at work, but now it seemed to Lydia that he was often moody and ill-tempered.

Little things upset him, and he reacted to minor irritations with uncharacteristic outbursts of bad language. Lydia knew it was not just her imagination because some of their friends also noticed the change in Ralph's personality.

As time went on, Lydia got more worried about her husband. Errands that he had accomplished without difficulty were now beyond him, and he no longer had the ability to concentrate on anything for any length of time.

When he tried to make a frame for a picture that Lydia had painted, it turned out the wrong size. Absurdly, he blamed Lydia for having used too large a piece of paper rather than himself for not having measured accurately.

Lydia also noticed that he had completely run out of energy and drive. He no longer suggested going on outings to do the sorts of things they had so enjoyed together in the past. Indeed, he did not really like leaving the house, and Lydia suspected that he became frightened and bewildered as soon as he was any distance from home. Several times neighbors had found him apparently lost on a nearby street and had to lead him home.

Even at home, Ralph showed little interest in what was going on. He appeared to read the newspaper at breakfast as he had always done, but Lydia noticed that later in the day he had no recollection of any of the headlines. When old friends came to visit, he took little part in the conversation. Sometimes, in fact, he did not seem to know who they were.

Ralph's dementia began at an unusually young age, since it is rare in people under the age of 70. But his decline illustrates many of the changes in personality and mental functions that are common in the early stages of this condition. It also shows the striking difference between the very common memory lapses that come with aging and the devastating impact of dementia. Memory lapses are embarrassing and a nuisance, but the individual's personality and ability to solve the problems of everyday life remain the same.

Dementia is quite different. Ralph's symptoms had been brought about by a disease that causes deterioration of almost every function of the brain.

## Key Points

- People often worry that memory problems are a sign of dementia.
- Most memory lapses are not caused by dementia.
- Dementia is a disease affecting memory, personality, and the ability to function in everyday life.

# What is dementia?

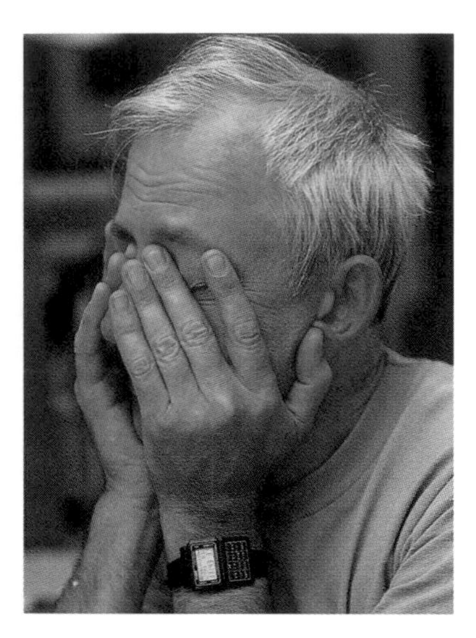

PROBLEMS OF DEMENTIA
*In the later stages of dementia, the symptoms include disorientation, personality changes, and anxiety.*

*Dementia is a term used by doctors to describe a progressive deterioration of mental powers accompanied by changes in behavior and personality.*

The story we told about Ralph in the last chapter illustrates some of the changes that are most frequently seen in someone who is suffering from the early stages of dementia. Individuals differ, of course, in the way they respond to a disease. Depending on age, the sort of people they are, and their physical health, the symptoms may vary a little between one person and another.

## WHAT ARE THE SYMPTOMS?

The symptoms of dementia include memory loss, personality changes, disorientation, inability to perform daily routine activities, and difficulty communicating.

### MEMORY LOSS

This is a common feature of dementia, and it is the memory of recent events that is affected first. The capacity to remember further back in time usually remains unaffected until the disease is at a more advanced stage. As we described earlier, in order to store a piece of information in our memory we first have to pay sufficient attention to register and absorb it so that we can recall it later. This ability to store recent information deteriorates because of the changes in the brain that occur in diseases such as Alzheimer's. In the early stages of dementia, this problem with short-term memory may not create too many difficulties; after all, many people find that their memories are less good as they get older. But, as the disease progresses, memory loss will become more severe. Sufferers may set out on an errand and then forget where they are going, or they may have a meal and later forget that they have eaten. In later stages, they may even forget the names of people close to them.

**Common Problems of Dementia**

- Deterioration of memory
- Disorientation
- Changes in personality and behavior
- Loss of practical everyday skills
- Difficulty in communicating

### DISORIENTATION

Closely connected to the failure of memory is the loss of the ability to orient oneself in direction or time. Many sufferers of dementia show signs of being disoriented, not knowing where they are or the current year, month, or day of the week. Sometimes they may get day and night confused, wanting to sleep during the day or go out in the middle of the night. You will remember from the last chapter that Ralph appeared bewildered when he was any distance from home. This deterioration in the ability to find one's way around becomes more marked as the disease advances. Sufferers may become more likely to wander away from home and get lost, which can pose a particular problem for those caring for them. In the later stages of the illness, they may have problems finding their way around their own home.

## Personality and Behavioral Changes

Some sufferers' personalities seem to remain much as they were before the onset of the disease, but others may show quite striking changes. Social withdrawal and a loss of interest in usual activities are common. People with dementia may experience formerly uncharacteristic mood swings, or some underlying part of their personality may become much more pronounced. They may develop a tendency toward spitefulness or anxiety. Some people seem to undergo drastic alterations in personality, changing perhaps from being gentle and placid most of the time into a person prone to outbursts of temper and aggression.

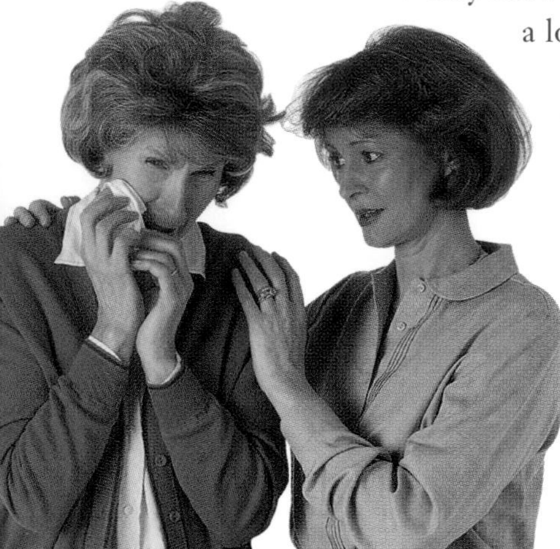

Emotional Outbursts *People with dementia often experience sudden, unpredictable mood changes. They may become anxious, distressed, or aggressive.*

As the disease progresses, many sufferers start to behave in ways that are socially unacceptable and may do or say things that would once have seemed totally inappropriate for them.

## Loss of Practical Skills

In the last chapter, we saw that Ralph lost the ability to perform everyday tasks and found it hard to concentrate for any length of time. This is one of the features of dementia. Sufferers have difficulty performing activities that they used to manage easily, such as driving, cooking, and, as the disease gets worse, even washing or dressing.

## Difficulties in Communication

In the early stages of dementia, people may have difficulty finding the correct words to use when speaking. This makes it harder to engage in complicated conversations, and taking phone messages can be a problem. Later they may be unable to finish sentences, often wandering to another subject, or they may repeat words over and over again. Reading and writing may also be affected.

It becomes even more difficult to find the right word when speaking as the disease progresses, and, since powers of comprehension also decline, conversation becomes increasingly difficult.

Using nonverbal forms of communication such as touch and facial expression become very important in caring for people in the later stages of dementia.

## Causes of Dementia

A number of diseases can produce the symptoms of dementia, and it is important to find out which of these is the cause. Some can be treated successfully, but there are others for which little can be done.

### Alzheimer's Disease

Alzheimer's disease is the most common cause of dementia in elderly people living in the US. In a very few cases, the disease occurs because of a defective gene, and several members of a family may be affected. However, this is an unusual reason for developing Alzheimer's disease, and most cases are not caused by this genetic abnormality. Scientists have not yet discovered the cause of the much more common form, which does not run in families. An enormous amount of research is being devoted to Alzheimer's disease. Some recent advances and current theories are described on pages 66–67.

Scientists have also been studying what happens to the nerve cells in the brains of sufferers. When a powerful microscope is used to look at a thin slice of brain from a patient with Alzheimer's disease, two features that are not present in the brains of people who do not have the disease can be seen: senile plaques and neurofibrillary tangles. The plaque is an accumulation of an abnormal protein, amyloid. One theory regarding the cause of Alzheimer's disease suggests that this plaque forms because the processes that normally operate to clear away this protein have become defective. Neurofibrillary tangles are skeins of another abnormal protein, but the tangle is found inside the nerve cells. The reason why the tangles develop is not known, but the normal processing of protein by the cell seems to be disrupted. These tangles choke the nerve cells and prevent them from working properly.

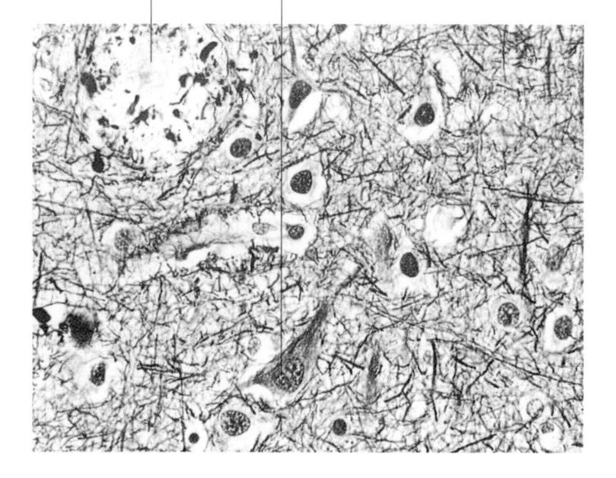


DISEASED BRAIN
*This micrograph of human brain tissue shows two characteristic features of Alzheimer's disease, senile plaques and neurofibrillary tangles.*

## LEWY BODY DEMENTIA

This type of dementia is characterized by distinct microscopic inclusions (Lewy bodies) seen in many areas of the brain like those seen in Parkinson's disease. Patients with Lewy body dementia suffer gradual onset of confusion often accompanied by hallucinations, delusions, and paranoia. The movement problems and rigidity of Parkinson's disease may precede or follow onset of these symptoms. Cognitive function, level of alertness, and degree of confusion can fluctuate in the early stages of the disease.

## FRONTAL LOBE DEMENTIA

This is a relatively common type of dementia characterized by degeneration of tissue in the frontal and part of the temporal lobes of the brain, which is visible on MRI scanning. Microscopic examination of the brain does not show the plaques and tangles seem in Alzheimer's disease. Patients experience changes in personality and behavior out of proportion to memory loss, sometimes resulting in alternating apathy and hyperactivity.

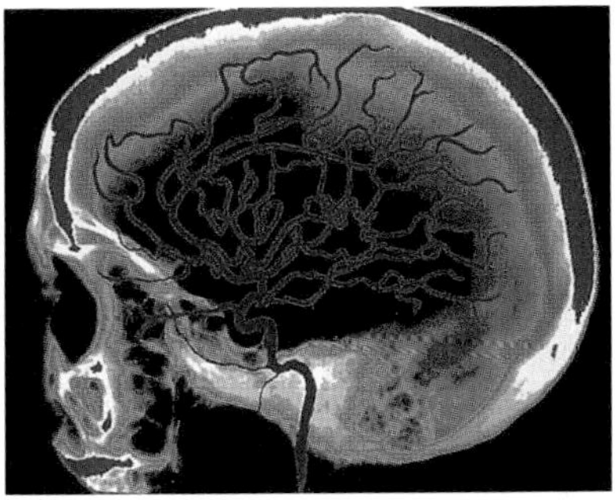

THE BRAIN'S BLOOD SUPPLY
*This angiogram of a human head shows the branching of one of the four arteries that supply blood to the brain.*

### VASCULAR DEMENTIA

Almost every part of the body needs blood because it carries oxygen and nutrients to the tissues and takes away carbon dioxide and other waste products. The brain is no exception. It is a very active organ that is richly supplied with blood through a dense network of many millions

## The Effect of Strokes on Brain Tissue

In vascular dementia, the effects of many small or large strokes accumulate, causing progressive damage to widespread areas of brain tissue where blood vessels have become blocked.

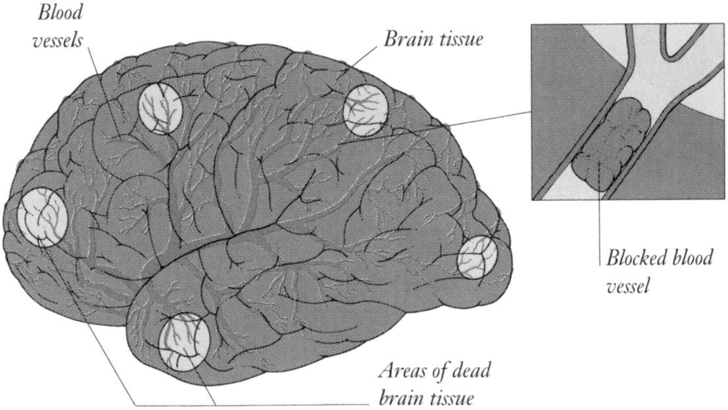

## Possible Causes of Dementia

*Dementia can arise from a number of different causes, the most common of which are listed below.*

- Alzheimer's disease
- Dementia with Lewy bodies
- Frontal dementia
- Vascular dementia
- Depression associated with dementia

Reversible causes of dementia:

- Vitamin $B_{12}$ deficiency
- Underactive thyroid
- Drug interactions
- Hereditary diseases of the nervous system
- Delayed effects of repeated injury

of tiny blood vessels. If some of them become blocked, they can no longer deliver blood. This is what happens when someone has a small stroke. The areas of the brain that were previously supplied by these blood vessels are deprived of oxygen, and some of the nerve cells die. An area of tissue that has died from lack of oxygen is called an infarct.

Widespread disease of small blood vessels can lead to the appearance of many tiny infarcts throughout the brain. Although each infarct is very small, the cumulative effect will disrupt normal brain functions. Sometimes this form is called multi-infarct dementia. Multi-infarct, or vascular, dementia is quite uncommon despite the relative frequency of strokes.

Our blood vessels tend to get narrower as we age. The process is somewhat similar to the buildup of mineral deposits in water pipes. However, disease of the small blood vessels is particularly common in people who have had high blood pressure for a long period of time, and this condition may be made worse by smoking.

### OTHER CAUSES OF DEMENTIA

The list of causes in the box above shows that dementia can occur for many reasons.

Sometimes the symptoms of dementia arise because of a metabolic or hormonal disturbance. For example, vitamin $B_{12}$ deficiency, an underactive thyroid, or, rarely, an adverse reaction to drug treatments can upset the balance of salts and chemicals in the blood and brain. If the dementia is caused by one of these, it can usually be treated successfully.

A large number of hereditary diseases can also cause dementia. Fortunately, they are all very rare.

Repeated head injuries, such as those suffered by professional boxers, sometimes result in the later development of a form of dementia.

In some cases, both the features of Alzheimer's disease and many tiny infarcts are found in the brain of someone who has died from dementia. Such people are said to have suffered from a mixed dementia.

To find out more about Alzheimer's disease, vascular dementia, or other rarer causes of dementia, see Further reading on page 75 for some books that may be helpful.

SEEING A DOCTOR
*If you suspect that someone you know is suffering from dementia, you should encourage him or her to seek an early diagnosis from a doctor.*

## WHAT SHOULD YOU DO?

If you are concerned that you, or someone close to you, are showing the symptoms just described, you should seek medical advice. There are several reasons why you should take action sooner rather than later. First, it can be difficult to diagnose dementia correctly. The symptoms that are worrying you may have another cause. One illness that often produces symptoms very similar to those of dementia, particularly in elderly people, is depression. You probably think of depression in terms of feeling both low in spirits and pessimistic about the future, but clinical depression involves much more than the temporary gloominess that we all feel occasionally. People suffering from severe depression may show so much difficulty with memory and concentration and such a loss of interest in their surroundings that they may appear to be suffering from dementia. It is especially important to recognize this because it usually can be successfully treated.

A second reason for talking to your doctor is that some other illnesses that produce symptoms of dementia can be cured, and it is important to diagnose them as early as possible. Even if the condition is incurable, treatment may be available that will prevent the symptoms from getting worse. Finally, if it does turn out to be a form of dementia for which there is no treatment, there is still much that can be offered in the way of practical help and support to improve the quality of life of sufferers and to ease the burden of those who care for them.

## KEY POINTS

- The symptoms of dementia include severe memory loss, disorientation, difficulties in communication, personality changes, and alterations in usual behavior.
- Dementia can arise from a number of different causes, including Alzheimer's disease, vascular disease, and even depression.
- Medical help should be sought as soon as possible.

# What will your doctor do?

*If you are worried about your own mental functions or are concerned that someone close to you is developing signs of dementia, you should consult your doctor right away.*

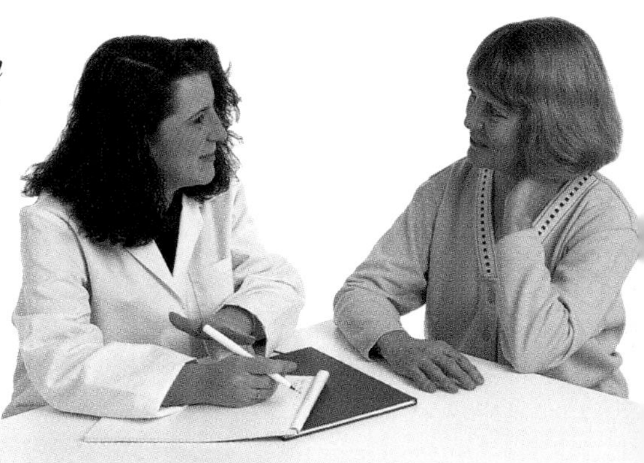

Here we explain how your doctor is likely to approach the problem, following Ralph and Lydia's story as an example. This will help you be prepared for the type of questions that you will be asked. We also describe briefly some of the tests that your doctor may feel are necessary and explain the reason for doing each of them.

GETTING A DIAGNOSIS
*If you are the caregiver of a person with suspected dementia, your doctor will want a detailed account from you of the sufferer's recent behavior.*

## ASSESSING THE HISTORY

Let us imagine that Lydia has persuaded Ralph to consult a doctor. They make an appointment to see his doctor, Dr. Elizabeth Garrett, and Lydia plans to go with her husband. To make a diagnosis, Dr. Garrett will need a detailed account of what has been happening to Ralph over the past few months. Since Ralph is often rather confused, it will be up to Lydia to provide reliable information. Although people often think that doctors make their diagnoses only from the results of medical tests such as X-rays or laboratory blood tests, the first and most crucial step is actually obtaining a clear description of the illness from the patient or a reliable witness. Tests come later and are used to confirm the doctor's clinical judgment or to help distinguish among a small number of possible causes of the illness. Lydia's story of the changes that have occurred in Ralph will be the first and most important clue in finding out what is wrong. By talking to Lydia as well as Ralph, Dr. Garrett will gain a fuller picture of the situation. The doctor will want to know:

- Whether any other members of Ralph's family have suffered from a disease of the nervous system.
- Details of Ralph's past illnesses, if any, although she may already have a record of this.
- Whether Ralph is taking medication, either prescribed for him by a doctor or bought over the counter at the pharmacy. Sometimes the wrong dose of a drug or a mixture of drugs can produce a confused state of mind that resembles dementia.

Dr. Garrett will also probably:

- Take Ralph's blood pressure.
- Conduct a full physical examination, paying particular attention to nervous system function.
- Perform various tests of mental performance. These will not be alarming to Ralph but will allow her to assess Ralph's memory and problem-solving abilities to confirm Lydia's story and assess the extent of Ralph's mental deterioration.

Depending on what Dr. Garrett finds, she may decide to perform some additional tests herself or she may arrange for Ralph to see a specialist who has expert knowledge of dementia and experience in treating it and its associated problems.

## REFERRALS TO SPECIALISTS

The availability of specialists varies from one part of the country to another. The type of specialist to whom a doctor refers a patient with suspected dementia will depend not only on what services are available in that particular area but also on characteristics of the patient such as age and the nature of the symptoms.

### THE CLINICAL PSYCHOLOGIST

It is often helpful if a clinical psychologist assesses someone with suspected dementia, since he or she is trained to assess memory, learning ability, and other mental functions. During an interview lasting about an hour, he or she will administer a number of tests. The results will provide a more detailed picture of the patient's mental abilities and difficulties.

### THE NEUROLOGIST

Neurologists are doctors who specialize in disorders that affect the brain and other parts of the nervous system. They treat patients with conditions such as Parkinson's disease, epilepsy, multiple sclerosis, and migraine. These patients often need brain scans as well as other tests that can be interpreted best by a neurologist.

If Dr. Garrett suspects that Ralph's symptoms are caused by a disease of the brain, she might refer him to a neurologist for a consultation and, if it is necessary, further investigation.

## THE GERIATRICIAN

Geriatricians specialize in the diseases and illnesses of the elderly. Failure of memory and deterioration of mental functions are quite common in older people, and geriatricians are expert at investigating the underlying cause of these mental changes.

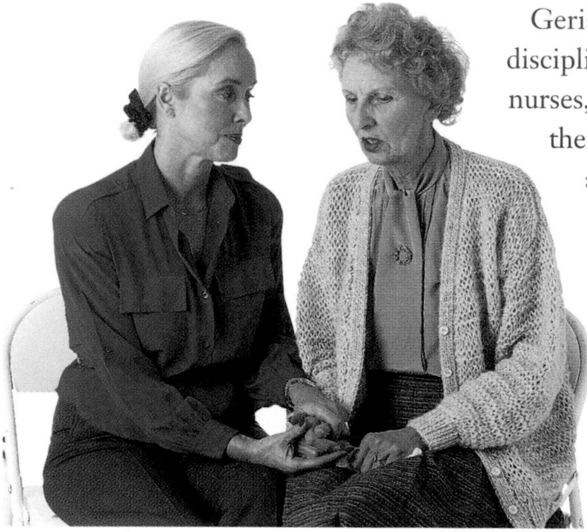

Geriatricians often utilize a multi-disciplinary team that is composed of nurses, occupational therapists, physical therapists, psychiatrists, nutritionists, and other specialists, as well as social workers, and they have particular expertise in arranging support for elderly people living at home.

HOME VISITS
*A geriatrician will often make home visits to assess the mental and physical capabilities of a patient.*

## THE PSYCHIATRIST

Psychiatrists are doctors who specialize in diagnosing and treating a wide range of mental health problems. Their assessment of a patient can be particularly helpful in those cases in which severe depression may be causing symptoms similar to those of dementia, making diagnosis difficult, or if behavioral problems associated with the dementia become difficult to manage.

## THE GERIATRIC PSYCHIATRIST

Geriatric psychiatrists are psychiatrists who specialize in the mental health problems of the elderly. They have special experience in diagnosing dementia, advising on the problems associated with the disease, and coordinating medical and social services to help look after sufferers.

## Tests and Investigations

There are a number of tests designed primarily to identify possible medical causes of mental dysfunction, such as hormone disturbances, chest infection, heart or lung disorders, and brain tumor.

### Blood Tests

In some cases, a deterioration in mental functioning can be the result of a disturbance in the body's metabolism or of an imbalance in the hormones that are circulating in the bloodstream. Analysis of a blood sample in the laboratory allows such a disturbance or imbalance to be detected. Laboratory analysis may be complicated, however, because accurate measurements have to be made of very small amounts of chemicals and hormones. Sometimes it may take a week or two before the results are sent back to the doctor who requested the tests. However, from the patient's point of view, these tests are easy and nearly painless. A small amount of blood is removed from a vein at the elbow or in the back of the hand and stored in a special tube until the laboratory is ready to perform the analysis. All the patient has to do is wait for the results.

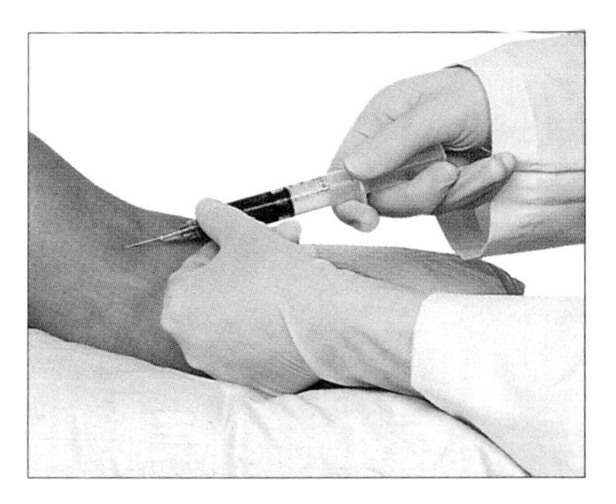

Taking Blood
*A blood sample will reveal the presence of any hormonal or metabolic imbalances in the body's system that could cause mental dysfunction.*

### CT and MRI Brain Scans

The letters CT stand for computerized tomography, a sophisticated type of X-ray that allows the brain to be visualized in great detail. The letters MRI stand for magnetic resonance imaging, a type of scan that uses magnetic fields to take a picture of the brain.

The person undergoing this test lies on a table with his or her head inside a circular hole, around which is the scanning equipment. The scanner produces a series of pictures showing cross sections of the brain at different levels, enabling the doctor to see whether there are any abnormalities that might be causing the symptoms.

### X-rays

X-rays of the chest may be performed to determine whether a chest infection or a heart or lung disorder might be contributing to the deterioration in the patient's mental functions.

Chest X-ray
*Ralph was sent to the hospital for a chest X-ray so that the doctor could rule out a disorder of the heart or lungs as the cause of his mental deterioration.*

## What Happens Next?

Once all the necessary tests and investigations have been conducted, the results will be sent to Dr. Garrett. If she referred Ralph to a specialist, he or she will write to Dr. Garrett, giving her the results of Ralph's tests, an assessment of his condition, and perhaps recommendations about treatment. It may take several months and perhaps several hospital visits before a definite diagnosis can be made.

Presently, there is no simple test that can show whether a person is definitely suffering from a progressive form of dementia, such as Alzheimer's disease. This diagnosis can be made only when all other possible causes of the symptoms have been eliminated.

When the tests and assessments have been completed, Lydia and Ralph will be able to go back either to Dr. Garrett or to the specialist to discuss the results and to plan how to deal with Ralph's condition.

## KEY POINTS

- The caregiver of a person who is suspected of having dementia will be asked about the patient's recent behavior.
- The doctor will perform a physical examination and a number of mental performance tests to help him or her make a diagnosis.
- The patient may be referred to a specialist.

# The emotional impact

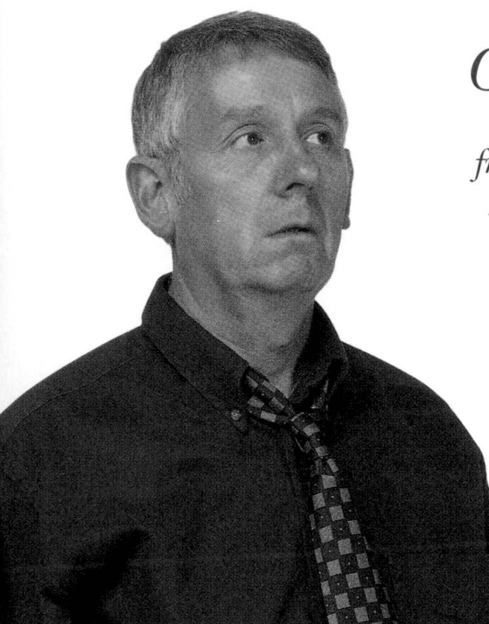

*Coming to terms with the fact that a member of your family is suffering from a progressive form of dementia, such as Alzheimer's disease, is very difficult. It is hard enough in the early stages to cope with the shock of the diagnosis and the changes that are already noticeable in the sufferer.*

LOSING SOMEONE
*As a person's mental capabilities worsen, friends and family will feel a deepening sense of grief as the person they knew is gradually lost to them.*

As the patient's illness progresses and the symptoms worsen, you will have to adjust to new signs of deterioration. People who care for someone with a chronic dementing illness need a great deal of support to help them deal with the powerful emotions that their sad predicament is bound to elicit. It is very important, if you are in such an unfortunate position, to recognize your own feelings and to realize that you will need emotional support from others. Far from being selfish, this will help you cope more effectively.

In this chapter, we describe some of the feelings that you may experience and offer some advice.

## SENSE OF LOSS

When someone close to you is diagnosed with dementia, you are bound to feel grief. The changes that the disease brings about in the sufferer's personality and behavior and his or her increasing inability to live a normal life arouse emotions similar to those experienced in bereavement. You will have to cope with feelings of distress and sadness at the loss of companionship; you are losing someone with whom you shared concerns and joys; and you may also be losing a sexual partner. This sense of grief will be heightened as you gradually understand the implications of the diagnosis. Coming to terms with your own feelings while having to look after the sufferer is a double burden.

What should you do? Sharing your concerns and feelings with family and friends can help you accept the situation and perhaps ease the sense of loss. Your doctor will be able to offer you psychological support and to refer you for counseling if you think it would help. Meeting other people who are in the same situation is another way of getting psychological help. There are support groups for caregivers in most parts of the country and there should be one located near you. Some of these are independent local caregivers groups, while others are run by national organizations. The Alzheimer's Association specializes in the needs of caregivers looking after people with all kinds of dementia. The National Caregiving Foundation (see Useful addresses, p.76) is also involved with support groups for the caregivers of dementia sufferers.

Addresses and telephone numbers for some of these organizations are included in Useful addresses. If there is no support group in your area, perhaps you could start one. Your doctor or nurse will probably be able to put you in touch with other families, and you could put up a notice in your physician's office or local library asking people who are interested to contact you.

## ANGER

It is natural to feel angry and resentful – angry that such a terrible thing has happened, angry perhaps that other members of the family don't help enough, and resentful that the future you had looked forward to has changed. In addition, you will have to deal with the daily exasperations and irritations of looking after the sufferer. People with dementia behave in ways that may make them extremely hard to live with.

Many people fail to recognize their anger or are afraid to express it. They may pretend to themselves that they are not really angry. Perhaps they are ashamed to be angry with someone who is ill. However, denying or bottling up these feelings of anger is not a good idea. Unless it is recognized and expressed, anger will lead to bitterness and resentment, which will only make it harder to cope with daily life.

One way of handling these feelings is to find ways to express them. Talk to other people about your irritation and anger. Other caregivers will know what you are going through, and discussing your feelings with them will help you cope better.

## GUILT

Guilt is also a common emotional reaction. When the disease is first diagnosed, it is natural to look for some explanation for what has happened. Sometimes people feel that perhaps something they did or failed to do caused the illness. If you have worries like this, it may be helpful to learn more about the disease and to discuss your concerns with your doctor.

Feeling embarrassed or even disgusted by the sufferer's behavior, losing your temper, wishing someone else could take on the caregiving responsibility, or taking care of someone to whom one has never been close can all produce feelings of guilt.

You may feel resentful and uncomfortable about taking on tasks that were normally the responsibility of the sufferer, and this too can cause guilt feelings. Caring for someone with dementia can sometimes involve a reversal of roles. You may be in a position of behaving like a parent to your mother or father. The assistance that sufferers need may be like that required by a small child of its parents, such as help with feeding and washing. It can be hard to adjust to this exchange of roles.

Most of us find it hard to accept that we cannot always live up to our own expectations or the expectations of others. It is important to be aware of your feelings, to try to assess the situation realistically, and not to expect too much of yourself. You may reach a stage at which you feel that the difficulties and stresses that caring for a demented person imposes on you and other family members are too great, and that the time has come to arrange for long-term residential care of the sufferer. This decision may produce a sense of relief as the burden is lifted, but also intense feelings of guilt. Talking things over with others may help. Realizing that such feelings are common and discussing how other people have coped will help you keep guilt feelings in proper perspective.

REVERSED ROLES
*You may find yourself helping a parent or grandparent with everyday practical matters, such as getting dressed, in much the same way that he or she once helped you as a child.*

## EMBARRASSMENT

One of the early effects of dementia is a loss of sensitivity to other people in social situations. The skills that are needed to maintain relationships are often among the first to disappear. Sufferers may lose the judgment necessary to behave or speak appropriately. It may become embarrassing to take them out, especially because strangers often do not understand what is happening. One way of dealing with this is to share your experiences with other caregivers.

Learning how others manage in similar situations will help you handle such problems with greater aplomb and less embarrassment and even to laugh about them. Explaining the illness to neighbors and friends can also ease your embarrassment because they will then understand the reason for the sufferer's behavior.

## LONELINESS

Being a caregiver is a lonely experience. The pressures of looking after a demented person make it difficult to maintain social activities. You may feel very much alone if the sufferer is the person with whom you used to share everything. Since loneliness can make it harder to solve the problems of everyday life, it is important not to let caring for the sufferer prevent you from devoting time to your own needs.

Make arrangements to share the caregiving so that you can spend time with family and friends or go to meetings and support groups for caregivers, such as those run by the Alzheimer's Association. Talking to other people in the same situation who understand your feelings can provide both support and friendship. Make some time for yourself to do things you enjoy.

## KEY POINTS

- It is extremely difficult to come to terms with the fact that someone close to you is deteriorating mentally.
- Emotional reactions to the diagnosis of dementia include a sense of loss, feelings of anger and guilt, embarrassment, and loneliness.

# Who can help?

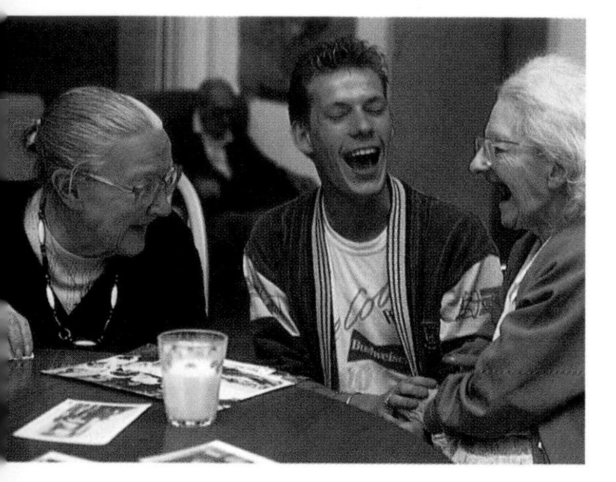

*If you are caring for someone with dementia, you are likely to need a good deal of practical support. The sufferer will find it increasingly hard to cope with everyday life, and you will not be able to provide all the assistance needed without help.*

USING DAY CARE
*Short-term relief, such as that provided by day care centers, can give a welcome break to both the patient and the caregiver.*

Unfortunately, it can sometimes be difficult to find information on the different types of help that are available. You may need to be persistent in your inquiries. Your doctor is likely to be a good source of information, but you should also talk to other caregivers. In this chapter, we discuss the kind of help that you will need, whether from family or from outside sources, such as Medicare, local social service agencies, and volunteer organizations.

## FAMILY AND FRIENDS

Families are a very important source of practical help and support. In some instances, it is possible to share the responsibility of caregiving. A brother and sister, for example, might take turns looking after their father, or one member of the family may make a regular commitment to look after the sufferer while the caregiver takes a respite. If, for a variety of reasons, it is not possible for the regular caregiver to share the burden of care with other members of the family, friends may well be happy to offer practical help as well as a sympathetic ear. They may be able to visit with the sufferer while the caregiver runs an errand.

## SPECIALIST NURSES

Many other sources of practical support can be organized by your doctor, including visiting nurses and community psychiatric nurses.

These nurses understand the practical difficulties of caring for a demented person at home. They can advise you whether any changes in the person's health need to be reported to your doctor and can teach you how best to overcome some of the practical problems of caregiving, such as bathing, eating problems, difficult behavior, incontinence, and giving medication.

The nurse can also provide help if the sufferer is frail and bedridden or needs a great deal of assistance in bathing, dressing, or getting to bed.

## OCCUPATIONAL AND PHYSICAL THERAPISTS

Your family doctor and the specialist can make arrangements for an occupational or physical therapist to visit the patient. They can advise on and arrange for aids and adaptations, such as hand rails, raised toilet seats, adapted cutlery, feeding aids, and devices that make dressing easier. They will also be able to advise you on eligibility for financial aid for major adaptations such as shower installations and wheelchair ramps.

## HELP IN THE HOME

Your local social service agency may be able to arrange for a home health aide to visit for several hours a week. An aide can provide practical help with housework, cleaning, laundry, and shopping and may also be able to assist with the personal care of the sufferer. Meals-on-wheels services exist in most areas. They provide a hot meal delivered to the house on certain days of the week. This is useful for sufferers who are still able to live alone. Your local area agency on aging (see Useful addresses, p.76) or social service agency will be able to give you more details.

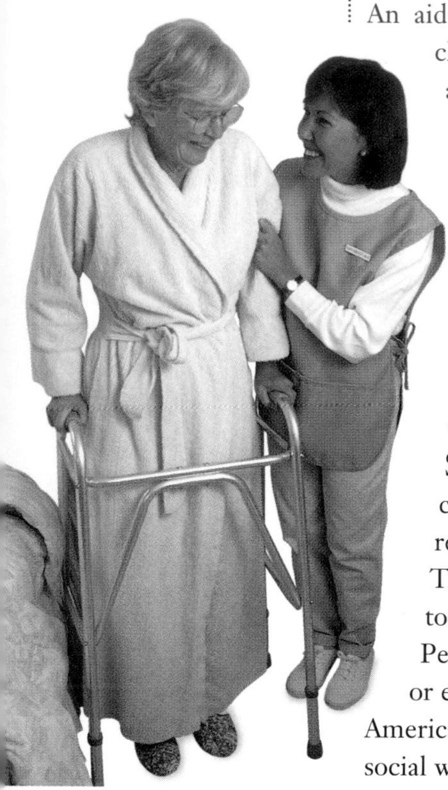

HELP IN THE HOME
*Outside caregivers such as home health aides can act as a source of both practical help and emotional support.*

## FINANCIAL HELP

Since caring for someone with dementia can be costly, it is important to make sure that you are receiving all the financial help that is available. There are a number of benefits and allowances to which you and the sufferer may be entitled. People with dementia may qualify for tax credits or extensions on state and federal income taxes. The American Bar Association, a local senior center, or a social worker can advise you of your eligibility and how to claim these benefits. If you are caring for a relative, you are entitled under the Family and Medical Leave Act of 1993 to up to 12 weeks of unpaid, job-protected leave. There are also many local programs that provide some form of financial assistance to family caregivers.

## SHORT-TERM RELIEF

One very important way to obtain help with the care of a demented person is to arrange for him or her to be cared for away from home for part of each day. This provides short-term relief for the main caregiver and may enable him or her to continue working part-time or to take care of other necessities of life. Your social worker or the local area agency on aging may be the best source of information on what is available in your area. Day care centers, which may be run either by local authorities or volunteer organizations, can provide recreational and social activities, lunch, and transportation to and from home. Some day care centers cater specifically to people with dementia. Psychogeriatric day hospitals offer medical assessment, social activities, and occupational therapy, but places in such hospitals are limited and are usually available only on a short-term basis.

Although day care centers provide the most common form of relief care, it may also be possible to arrange for someone to come to your home to care for the sufferer. Some volunteer agencies provide sitters for a few hours. Alternatively, local caregivers' support groups may arrange sitting services, with members taking turns so that everyone has an opportunity for time off. Private agencies can supply a care attendant or a nurse to look after the sufferer for longer periods, but this form of care is expensive.

If you want to go away on vacation or need a longer break from the burdens of caregiving, it may be possible to arrange residential care in a home or nursing facility. This respite care is provided specifically to allow caregivers a break. Alternatively, you could use one of the many private nursing and residential homes. Your doctor or local area agency on aging should be able to advise you about what is available in your area.

## KEY POINTS

- Practical and emotional support may come from family, friends, your doctor, local caregivers' groups, or a social service agency.
- Organizations that can help are listed in Useful addresses (see p.76).

# What can be done?

*We have already described the way in which your doctor will try to find out what is causing the symptoms of mental deterioration. Should the cause prove to be a metabolic disturbance, or a hormone or vitamin $B_{12}$ deficiency, your doctor will take steps to correct the problem, and there is a very good chance that the symptoms will improve.*

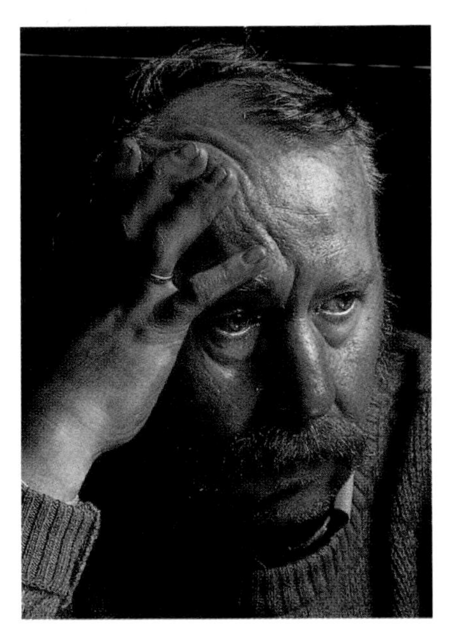

IMPROVING THE SYMPTOMS
*A doctor will be able to relieve the sufferer's symptoms if they are caused by a metabolic disturbance or a hormone or vitamin deficiency.*

What if it turns out that the symptoms are due to a progressive form of dementia such as Alzheimer's disease? Can anything be done? Unfortunately, no treatment is yet available that can cure Alzheimer's disease. A few drugs have been given to sufferers experimentally in trials to see whether they are effective in decreasing the severity of the symptoms and slowing the progression of the disease. Although some trials have suggested that some patients may benefit from taking drugs, other trials with other groups of patients have failed to confirm the results. There is also the disadvantage that some of these treatments carry a risk of quite serious side effects. Most of these drugs are still at the experimental stage and are not generally available because the hazards of taking them outweigh the potential benefits. Two new drugs that are now available by prescription in the US are tacrine and donepezil. Trials have shown that scores on some tests of mental functioning were slightly better in patients taking these drugs.

Not all patients respond to these treatments. Even when improvements do occur, they may not be great enough to have a worthwhile effect on patients' symptoms or day-to-day functioning.

Vascular dementia is another disease that, like Alzheimer's disease, causes dementia. It occurs when some of the small vessels that carry blood to the brain become blocked. The area of the brain supplied by a blocked blood vessel dies from lack of oxygen. By the time symptoms are noticeable, it is too late to try to unblock the vessel, but it is possible to try to prevent the condition from getting worse.

High blood pressure is one reason why blood vessels tend to get blocked, but this can be treated safely and effectively with drugs. Another possible cause of blood vessel blockage is an increased tendency of the blood to clot. It has been found fairly recently that a low dose of aspirin is very effective in counteracting this tendency. A small daily dose of aspirin is frequently advised. Unfortunately, however, these measures often do not change the outcome in someone who suffers from vascular dementia.

At the current time, most medical treatment of people suffering from dementia emphasizes control of the various problems that can make these people so difficult to care for. Effective treatments can be prescribed in order to reduce restlessness and agitation and improve mood and sleep patterns. However, these symptoms do not always require treatment with medication, and it may be better to approach the problem in other ways.

## Depression

It can sometimes be difficult to distinguish between the symptoms of severe depression and those of dementia. Correct diagnosis is very important because effective drugs are available to treat severe depression, but not dementia. Sometimes people with dementia may become quite depressed. They cry frequently, are withdrawn, and are unable to enjoy anything.

Treatment with antidepressant drugs improves the mood of such people, helps them sleep, and may lead to a reduction in behavioral problems. If you think the person you are caring for may be suffering from depression, talk to your doctor, who may decide to get an opinion from a psychiatrist or geriatric psychiatrist before prescribing treatment.

## Behavioral Problems

As the disease progresses, sufferers may behave in ways that those caring for them find both distressing and difficult to handle. People with dementia sometimes behave in a very aggressive manner, becoming verbally abusive or even physically violent. They may overreact to a slight setback and get frustrated, upset, or angry. They may also become agitated and restless, constantly moving around the house or wandering off for no apparent reason. Some sufferers lose their normal inhibitions and start behaving in socially unacceptable ways, such as removing their clothes in public.

If you are caring for someone with dementia, you may be able to deal with some of these behavioral problems by taking preventive measures. Take note of the sort of situations that are likely to trigger such reactions and work out ways of avoiding them. Maintaining a calm, familiar, and unstressful environment for the sufferer will help prevent outbursts of anger and distress.

You may be able to get advice on how best to deal with emotional and behavioral problems from a psychiatric nurse. Such nurses provide support for people with mental health problems and their families. Your doctor should be able to arrange this for you.

If levels of distress, agitation, and aggression are very high and do not respond to these simple measures, treatment with medication can be helpful. The drugs have a calming and sedating effect, but they may produce unwanted side effects. They can be prescribed only by a doctor, and they must be used under close medical supervision.

## KEY POINTS

- There is no cure yet available for Alzheimer's disease.
- Drugs designed to improve the symptoms are becoming available.
- The benefits of these new drugs seem to be modest.
- Treatment with various medications can help reduce agitation and improve mood if behavioral interventions are not effective.

# Why did it happen?

*Whenever a change in our lives is forced upon us, we want to know the reason for it. So it is easy to understand why a diagnosis of dementia in a family member often leads people to try to identify some event or factor that might have caused the disease.*

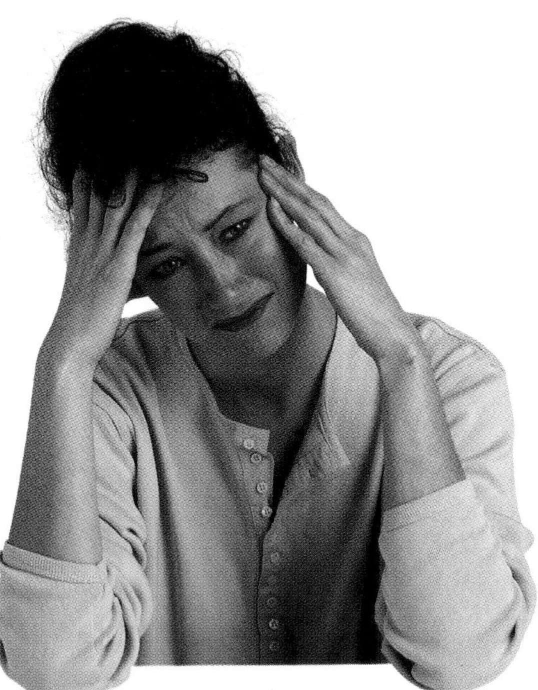

If, for example, the symptoms of dementia first became noticeable after moving or in the months following retirement, it would be tempting to conclude that the stresses and life changes that accompanied these events were somehow to blame for the onset of the disease.

BLAMING YOURSELF
*Many caregivers feel guilty, quite mistakenly, thinking that they may have done something to contribute to someone's dementia.*

## MISPLACED GUILT

Some people go further than this and believe that they themselves may be to blame for what happened. They worry that something they did or failed to do may have caused the disease or made the symptoms worse. It is all too easy to find yourself thinking, "If only I'd taken him to see the doctor sooner," "I should have taken more notice of the changes in him," or "I wish that I'd been more sympathetic."

It is very important not to blame yourself in this way. The symptoms of dementia appear so gradually that it is very hard to notice that something is wrong with someone you see every day. Friends and relatives who do not see the sufferer very often are in a much better position to recognize these gradual changes, and they are frequently the first to notice a deterioration.

## THE CAUSES OF DEMENTIA

The causes of Alzheimer's disease are as yet unknown, although there are several theories that are discussed later in this chapter. A little more is known about vascular dementia. But first, let us examine factors that do NOT cause dementia. A great deal of research is being carried out to learn more about the disease and why some individuals are susceptible to it. The results of this research show that many of the popular ideas about the causes of dementia are incorrect.

### WHAT NOT TO BLAME

- **Underuse of the brain** Many people believe that mental faculties deteriorate if they are not used enough. This is sometimes known as the "use it or lose it" theory. According to this view, old people are less likely to become demented if they remain mentally active and have lots of interests, but this is mistaken. Alzheimer's disease and other causes of dementia affect all sorts of people from all walks of life. There are many good reasons to make efforts to keep your mind alert after retirement, but doing so will not protect you from dementia.
- **Overuse of the brain** There is no evidence that "thinking too much" or working too hard can cause

dementia. You cannot damage or wear out your brain with mental activity.

- **Stressful life events** Dementia is not caused by sudden changes or stressful adverse events such as changing jobs, suffering bereavement, getting divorced, moving, being admitted to the hospital, or having accidents, although such events may indeed sometimes bring a hidden dementia to light. The sufferer may have been able to cope previously, but a sudden change or a stressful experience may prove too much, and the symptoms of dementia become noticeable for the first time. It may appear that the event has caused the dementia, but in fact the disease had already taken hold, and the event only made it more obvious.
- **Psychological problems** People who have suffered from anxiety or depression are sometimes thought to be more at risk of developing dementia, but there is no clear evidence that this is so. Depression is sometimes one of the symptoms in the early stages of dementia, and this may be why it has sometimes mistakenly been regarded as a cause of the disease.
- **Alcohol** Alcohol affects brain function at least in a temporary way, and it is perhaps not surprising that many people believe that heavy or prolonged drinking can lead to a loss of brain cells. Sometimes brain damage does occur in malnourished alcoholics, but this type of dementia is rare and is different from Alzheimer's disease or vascular dementia.
- **Smoking** It has been suggested that smoking may actually protect people from Alzheimer's disease, but as yet there is not a great deal of evidence to support this. However, smokers do seem to be more likely to develop vascular dementia.

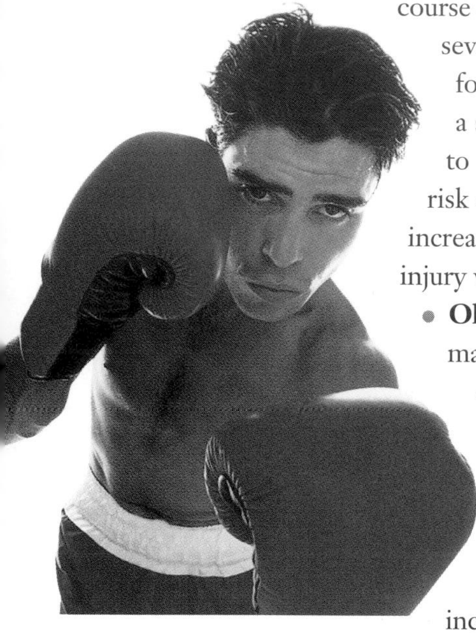

- **Head injury** Everyday mishaps, such as banging one's head on a kitchen cabinet, do not cause dementia, but certain groups of people, such as boxers, who in the course of their careers have been subjected to repeated severe blows to the head, do sometimes develop a form of dementia. Experts argue about whether a single violent injury to the head serious enough to result in loss of consciousness increases the risk of Alzheimer's disease. If it does, the risk is not increased very much. Most people who survive a head injury will not get Alzheimer's disease.
- **Old age** Dementia is not caused by old age, and the majority of elderly people do not develop it. However, like almost every other illness, dementia is more likely to occur in older people.

OCCUPATIONAL HAZARD
*Professional boxers who receive repeated blows to the head can suffer from a form of dementia.*

## ALZHEIMER'S DISEASE

There is major research into the origin of Alzheimer's disease under way, and explanations include genetic and environmental causes.

### GENETIC CAUSES

In a small proportion of the people who develop the disease at an unusually early age, Alzheimer's disease is genetic. In some of these families, a defective gene located on chromosome 21 has been identified as the cause of the disease. This explanation, however, is the exception rather than the rule. Only a very small percentage of the total number of cases of Alzheimer's disease can be attributed to this defective gene.

Recently, a genetic predisposition to the more common form of Alzheimer's disease that affects older people has been discovered. People who carry a particular form of the gene for apolipoprotein E are at increased risk. This gene contains the information that the body needs to make a protein that is important for the development and health of the brain. There are three variants of this protein. There is now good evidence that possessing one of these variants leads to a modest increase in the chances of developing Alzheimer's disease late in life. How this variant of apolipoprotein E acts to increase susceptibility to Alzheimer's disease is not yet understood.

### ENVIRONMENTAL CAUSES

A large number of environmental factors that might cause Alzheimer's disease have been investigated. They include foreign travel; type of occupation; use of chemicals, drugs, and medicines; tea and coffee drinking; a nd malnutrition. There also have been studies to find out whether people who have had surgery or general anesthesia or who have suffered from some other disease are more likely to develop Alzheimer's disease. The finger of suspicion does not point directly to any of these possibilities at present.

## VASCULAR DEMENTIA

This form of dementia has its origin not in the nerve cells of the brain but in disease of the small blood vessels that carry oxygen and fuel to this organ. One very important factor that leads to this blood vessel disease is high blood pressure. People whose blood pressure has been abnormally high for a number of years are more likely to develop vascular dementia.

Another factor that makes this type of dementia more likely is smoking, which increases the tendency

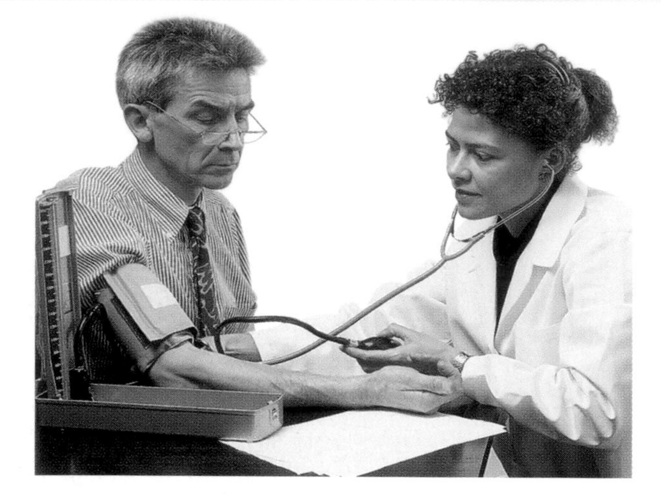

HIGH BLOOD PRESSURE
*It is important to have your blood pressure monitored by your doctor, because hypertension can increase the risk of tiny strokes in the brain that may cause vascular dementia.*

of the blood to clot. The combination of disease of the small blood vessels and blood that tends to clot too readily is dangerous. It is likely to lead to the blockage of blood vessels and damage to the areas of the brain normally supplied by the blocked vessels.

## KEY POINTS

- In a few cases, people have developed Alzheimer's disease because of a defective gene, but in most cases the cause of the disease is unknown.
- One significant cause of vascular dementia is high blood pressure.

# The future

*Alzheimer's disease or any other form of dementia is a personal tragedy for the sufferers and for those who love them and bear the burden of caring for them. It is a tragedy that is affecting more and more people.*

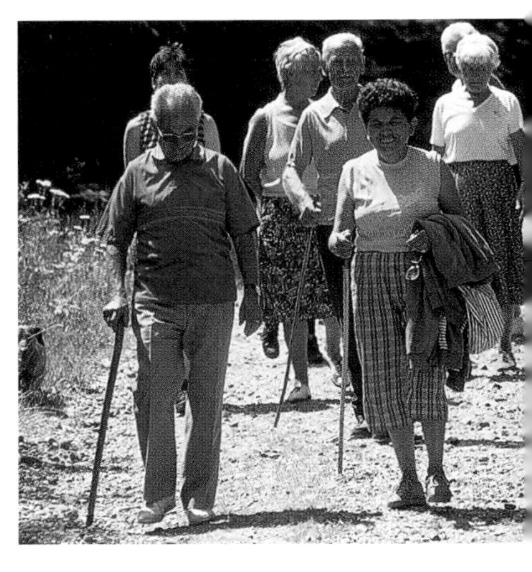

LIVING LONGER
*With the steady increase in life expectancy over recent decades comes an increase in the number of cases of diseases that affect the older generation, including dementia.*

Not very long ago, doctors believed that Alzheimer's disease and other conditions that cause dementia were quite rare. Today, everyone has heard of dementia, and many have had the sad experience of looking after a close relative suffering from some form of it. Why is this? One important reason is that the world's population is living longer.

## THE AGING POPULATION

At the beginning of the 20th century, the average life expectancy was about 50 years. Thanks to improved living conditions – better housing, better nutrition, and better medical care – an increasing proportion of each succeeding generation has survived into old age. The average life expectancy in the US today is now nearly 80 years. As a result of this improvement, as well as the fact that people have been having smaller families, the population has been growing older. In 1951, only 7 percent of the population was aged 65 and older, but by 1996 this had grown to 18 percent. This aging of the population means, of course, that there are many more cases of diseases that affect elderly people.

The population of the United States and of almost every other country in the world will continue to get older until well into the 21st century. We can therefore predict that dementia will become an even bigger problem as time goes on. Approximately 4 million Americans now have Alzheimer's disease. By the middle of the next century it is estimated that this will increase to 14 million unless a cure or prevention is found. Countries in the developing world, such as Brazil, Kenya, and Bangladesh, where populations are young and dementia is still a rare condition, will soon be faced with the same problem.

## RESEARCH INTO DEMENTIA

If you are looking after someone with dementia, you may feel very lonely. Perhaps it seems as if no one else cares much about what you are going through. This impression is quite wrong. There is a major medical research effort in all the countries of the western world into discovering the causes of Alzheimer's disease and the other diseases that lead to dementia. Equally important, scientists are working hard to develop successful treatments for dementia.

Let us look at what has been achieved so far and what we hope will happen in the future. If progress seems slow, you must remember that only 20 years ago dementia was not thought to be a significant medical problem and was low on the list of priorities for research. Since we knew very little about the condition then, researchers had to start almost from scratch.

One of their first tasks was to determine the extent of the problem. Epidemiologists – medical researchers who study the patterns of disease in the population – have conducted many surveys in different parts of the world, and, as a result, we have a fairly accurate idea of how frequently dementia occurs. This information was crucial in drawing attention to the scale of the problem and the urgency of studying the disease. Some of these surveys also provided clues about the causes of some of the diseases that result in dementia. For example, the results of several studies performed in North America and Britain suggested that Alzheimer's disease was more common where the drinking water contained small amounts of aluminum. Further studies, however, failed to confirm any link between aluminum and Alzheimer's disease.

In the laboratory, enormous strides have been made toward understanding the processes that go on inside the nerve cells of the brains of people affected by Alzheimer's disease. We now know that a protein molecule whose normal function is to join one cell to its neighbor accumulates in abnormally large quantities in the brains of Alzheimer's sufferers. It appears that the cellular machinery that breaks down this protein when it is no longer needed fails. If we can find out why it fails, it may be possible to do something about it.

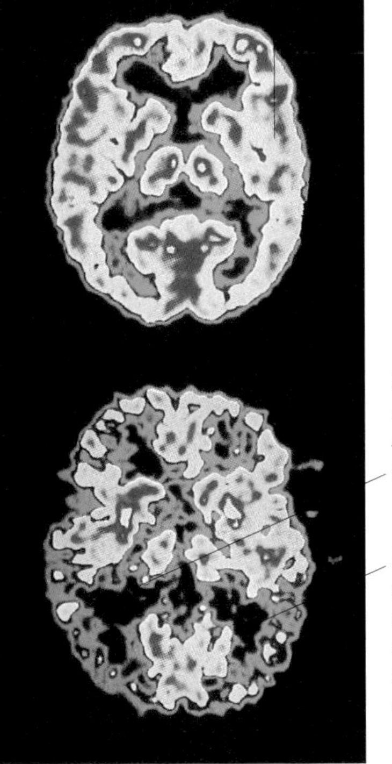


REDUCED BRAIN ACTIVITY
*Compared with a normal brain (top), a scan of one affected by Alzheimer's disease (bottom) shows a loss of brain material. Blue and black areas indicate low brain activity.*

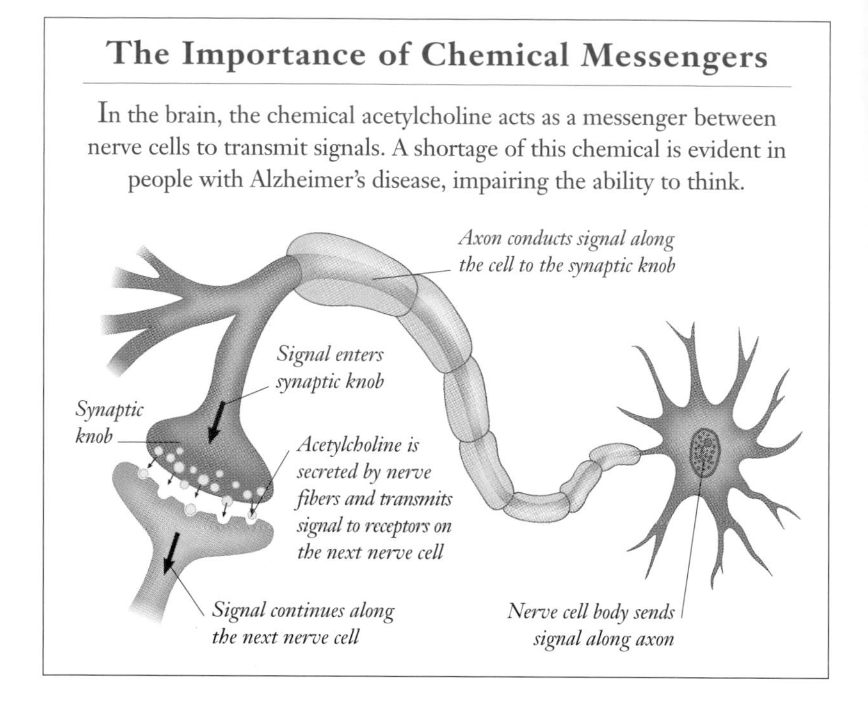


## The Importance of Chemical Messengers

In the brain, the chemical acetylcholine acts as a messenger between nerve cells to transmit signals. A shortage of this chemical is evident in people with Alzheimer's disease, impairing the ability to think.

Biochemists have discovered that levels of a chemical called acetylcholine are very low in some parts of the brain in people who have died with Alzheimer's disease.

Acetylcholine is one of the chemical messengers in the brain that allows one nerve cell to communicate with another. This discovery led to research to find drugs that raise the levels of acetylcholine such as donepezil and tacrine. It is hoped that replenishing stores of this chemical will partly restore brain function.

Geneticists, too, are working on the problem of dementia. An important discovery made a few years ago was that, in a small number of cases, Alzheimer's disease is caused by a defective gene. If geneticists can find out what the gene does under normal circumstances, we may gain a better understanding of what goes wrong in the disease.

## THE OUTLOOK

We do not yet know which of these lines of research will prove to be fruitful and which will not. We cannot predict where the next advance will come from, and it is important that investigation continues on a broad front. Finding out the causes of dementia and understanding what goes wrong inside the nerve cells of the brain is a very difficult task. Progress is slow, and, if you are looking after someone with dementia, we must warn you that advances will probably come too late to help you.

Some people who know or take care of a person with dementia decide to join one of the volunteer organizations mentioned earlier. These groups offer help and advice to sufferers and their families, and some also provide funding for scientists who are investigating the causes of dementia and trying to develop treatments. Individuals can help in a number of ways, whether by taking part in fund-raising activities or volunteering to help with home care services, transportation arrangements, or support groups. By getting involved in this way, people often feel that they have a chance to do something positive. It is one way in which good can come out of the tragedy that is dementia.

## KEY POINTS

- People are tending to live longer.
- In an aging population, the number of cases of diseases that affect the elderly, including Alzheimer's, is increasing.
- There is a major medical research effort taking place to discover the causes of Alzheimer's disease and other diseases that lead to dementia.

# Further reading


**Alzheimer's Disease and Dementia**

Davis, Helen D., and Michael P. Jensen
*Alzheimer's: The Answers You Need*
Forest Knolls, CA: Elder Books, 1998

Feil, Naomi
*The Validation Breakthrough: Simple Techniques for Communicating with People with "Alzheimer's-Type Dementia"*
Baltimore: Health Professionals Press, 1994

Gillick, Muriel R.
*Tangled Minds: Understanding Alzheimer's Disease and Other Dementias*
New York: Dutton, 1998

Mace, Nancy L., Peter V. Rabins, and Paul R. McHugh
*The 36-Hour Day: A Family Guide to Caring for Persons with Alzheimer Disease, Related Dementing Illnesses, and Memory Loss in Later Life*, 3rd ed.
Baltimore: Johns Hopkins University Press, 1999

Rabins, Peter V., Constantine G. Lyketsos, and Cynthia Steele
*Practical Dementia Care*
New York: Oxford University Press, 1999

**Memory**

Baddeley, Alan
*Your Memory: A User's Guide*, 2nd ed.
North Pomfred, VT: Trafalgar Square, 1996

Higbee, Kenneth L.
*Your Memory: How It Works and How to Improve It*, 2nd ed.
New York: Marlowe, 1996

Rupp, Rebecca
*Committed to Memory: How We Remember and Why We Forget*
New York: Crown, 1998

# Useful addresses

**Administration on Aging**
Online: www.aoa.dhhs.gov
330 Independence Avenue, SW
Washington, DC 20201
Tel: (800) 677-1116
Tel: (202) 619-0724
Fax: (202) 260-1012
The toll-free number gives you a link to the Eldercare Locator, which gives information on services for older people in their communities, including meals, transportation, legal services, and help for caregivers.

**Alzheimer's Association**
Online: www.alz.org
919 North Michigan Avenue
Chicago, IL 60611
Tel: (800) 272-3900
Tel: (312) 335-8700
Fax: (312) 335-1110

**Alzheimer's Disease Education and Referral Center National Institute of Aging**
Online: www.alzheimers.org
PO Box 8250
Silver Spring, MD 20907
Tel: (800) 438-4380
Fax: (301) 495-3334

**Family Caregiver Alliance**
Online: www.caregiver.com
425 Bush Street,
Suite 500
San Francisco, CA 94108
Tel: (415) 434-3388

**National Caregiving Foundation**
Online: www.ncoa.org
801 North Pitt Street
Alexandria, VA 22314
Tel: (703) 288-9300
Advises on all aspects of caregiving.

**National Council on Aging**
Online: www.ncoa.org
409 Third Street
Washington, DC 20024
Tel: (800) 424-9046

# Index

# Acknowledgments

PUBLISHER'S ACKNOWLEDGMENTS

Dorling Kindersley Publishing, Inc. would like to thank the following for their help and participation in this project:

**Managing Editor** Stephanie Jackson; **Managing Art Editor** Nigel Duffield; **Editorial Assistance** Janel Bragg, Mary Lindsay, Irene Pavitt, Jennifer Quasha, Design Revolution; **Design Assistance** Sarah Hall, Marianne Markham, Design Revolution, Chris Walker; **Production** Michelle Thomas, Elizabeth Cherry.

**Consultancy** Dr. Tony Smith, Dr. Sue Davidson; **Indexing** Indexing Specialists, Hove; **Administration** Christopher Gordon.

**Organizations** St. John's Ambulance, St. Andrew's Ambulance Organization, British Red Cross.

**Picture Research** Angela Anderson; **Picture Librarian** Charlotte Oster.

PICTURE CREDITS

The publisher would like to thank the following for their kind permission to reproduce their photographs. Every effort has been made to trace the copyright holders. Dorling Kindersley apologizes for any unintentional omissions and would be pleased, in any such cases, to add an acknowledgment in future editions.

**APM Studios** p.9; **Barnaby's Picture Library** p.13 (Micky White); **Robert Harding Picture Library** p.69; **Sally & Richard Greenhill Photo Library** p.3, p.32, p.54; **Science Photo Library** p.36, p.37 (CNRI), p.59 (Oscar Burnel/Latin Stock), p.71 (National Institute of Health); **Telegraph Color Library** p.12 (R. Chapple), p.20 (Bildagentur), p.56 (R. Chapple), p.66 (Stock Directory/VCL).